The Telling, The Listening

SAINT JULIAN PRESS

POETRY

Praise for ~ The Telling, The Listening

In this moving book, mostly unrhymed free verse lines recall the speaker's experience (sometimes as the generator) of unexpected moments of grace and reprieve during decades of practicing medicine. The poems follow a life given over to service: "I will love this midnight world. / I will love my calling. / I will love your need" (from "Night Call"). This doctor remembers her patients by name, suffers with them, and spins powerful poetry from that shared pain. When death comes to her patients, she greets it with dignity, turning off life's noisy, over-bright monitors and, in one stunning poem ("The ICU Nurse Sang"), keeping vigil with a night nurse who sings a lullaby. Read this book to remember that the doctors we expect to be gods are human, too—they feel fatigue, fear, and despair. Sometimes, they wear red silk next to their skin. Read it also for the pleasure of its well-wrought lines and to feel supported, or at least less alone, in your own experience of infirmity or pain.

—Rebecca Foust
ONLY (Four Way Books 2022)
& Marin County Poet Laureate Emerita.

In *The Telling, The Listening,* physician poet Catharine Clark-Sayles bleeds out lyrical narrative after narrative about delivering difficult news to patients, searching for what to say and what to do in a world with no final answers, only stories carried away from countless encounters at the intersection of entropy and the limits of medicine. But those stories—delivered with musical and gripping diction: a child's "bloodied rags of flesh…seen through the sniper scope," a "young man completely healthy until purple blotches / on his face doubled in a week, lungs whited out," "…the woman dying / in her eighty-ninth year—…there was a boy— / I let him kiss me once, but then he hit me / and held me down…"—these and scores more of the scarred and dying, treated by doctors that collect patient's pain and add it to their own, will teach readers how to negotiate with their own pain and existential angst, both on the page and in the stories they tell others and themselves.

—Terry Lucas
Dharma Rain

The Telling, The Listening by Catharine Clark-Sayles is amazing. This book tells of medical experiences she had as a military doctor and then as a California physician. The moving poems are not only about patients but also of her family, her loves, and even the disastrous fall she took several years ago while hiking. Her poetic work is skillful and detailed. When she couldn't hold a dying friend's hand because family members had both, she says she held on to one toe. Yes, her work is about some people who recover, yet many who will not. Throughout the book, Clark-Sayles projects her deeply moving empathy, but still the conviction that every life she treats is significant. In her poem "Words Beyond Words" she says: "True healing comes from stories: the telling, the listen. / "Tell me," I say and see your tears begin to glisten."

—Susan Terris
Familiar Sense

The stark yet compassionate words here spell out for us a very personal, inside view of the doctor-patient relationship: its harsh reality, weighted emotional conditions, and the personal impact of disease upon both doctor and patient. The guard is taken down, the wall broken, and there is a frank exchange of data and emotion that crosses over between doctor and patient, and now, to us, the reader of these well-crafted poems. When the poet is capable of writing lines like "no cure in pills; just nectar-drops of hope, a sweetness of belief," we know we are dealing with a clear-visioned teller of the way things are. We can trust this voice to take us to the heart of the matter.

—David Watts
Bedside Manners and *Having and Keeping*

The Telling,

The Listening

Poems

by

Catharine Clark-Sayles

SAINT JULIAN PRESS
HOUSTON

Published by
SAINT JULIAN PRESS, Inc.
2053 Cortlandt, Suite 200
Houston, Texas 77008

www.saintjulianpress.com

ISBN-13: 978-1-955194-18-1

Library of Congress Control Number: 2023940664

Cover Art: *cats sleeping on the rooftops*
Artist: Octavio Quintanilla

THIS BOOK IS DEDICATED TO THE DOCTORS, NURSES, AND PATIENTS WHO TAUGHT ME MEDICINE AND THE TEACHERS WHO TAUGHT ME POETRY. THERE ARE TOO MANY TO NAME, BUT EACH ONE IS WRITTEN IN MY HEART.

CONTENTS

III

"Listen to your patient; he is telling you the diagnosis."
—Sir William Osler, M.D.

"For the patient's story will come to you
like hunger, like thirst."
—Dr. John Stone, M.D. Cardiologist

The Telling, The Listening

I

Triage As It Is Taught

"Preserve the fighting strength" — the Army doctors' mission.
Cure only if resources will allow, the most badly broken—
label "expectant", set aside, morphine doses hash-
marked in black marker on the forehead

and if, hours later, after the repairable are straightened, sutured,
bandaged, the surgeons winnow through and set to salvage work—
some triaged back to live whatever sort of mangled life is left.

What We Carry

For Dr. Oskar

Your shoulders, lumpy and misshapen, are giving you pain.
I look at the X-ray on the wall, strange alignment and
rotations—
and ask how this came to be. In a soft voice you recite
facts: sixteen,
lines—you sent left, mothers and sisters sent right,
blue numbers inked on your arm, I have seen them and know—
in abstraction—the meaning, now you tell me about beatings,
of being hung by your wrists with hands tied behind your back,
then a march through snow, how the ones who fell were shot.
You tell me all this gently and I hear the end of the story—
American POWs dressed you in bits of their uniforms, insisted
you were one of them, how they helped you later to New York,
to a life of poet, doctor, and scholar. Last month— a grandson's
bar mitzvah.
You say you don't really believe in God, but your grandson does
and you are proud of that. I struggle for balance, my careful
objective distance smashed on the walls of your story,
you apologize for tears in my eyes. But if you can bear to love
children, love a woman for fifty-seven years, love gardens,
pear trees
you grafted yourself, love the iambic beat of a poem;
if you can bear to live, how can I not bear to carry your story?

The PTSD Clinic

How does a doctor heal fear-memory: the click of a stepped-on mine,
bloodied rags of flesh, once a child, seen through the sniper scope,
revved engine of the suicide bomber aimed at the guarded gate,
smell of gunpowder and singed flesh, a muzzle flash from a broken
window overhead, the grit of sand in every crease, days old sweat
salt crust
and stink, mortars screaming down as the night sky lights red
with flares.

The past, like sucking sand pulls a human back to moments
of vast inhumanity, makes them an amber-trapped fly—
its frantic buzzing slows and stills, settles in to stay forever
in that moment as the body moves through whatever is required,
finding reasons to survive, until the count of reason dwindles to zero
and the wounded animal of the body is put down.

The pills I give seldom still anxiety, and pain is only dulled,
sleep eludes and there are no pills for nightmares that bleed
into a sleep-starved day and dreams don't run from guns and knives
no matter how strong the need for arms to face the grocery store,
the trips for gas and liquor, the mandatory anger management class.

Once in an Army hospital, in Baghdad by the Bay with a panoramic
view of the city, a booming pass by Blue Angels jets in practice
formations
for a show to delight the Fleet Week crowds had half a dozen men
dive to the floor, belly-crawling under beds, hands over ears,
screaming while the nurses ran for tranquilizers.

Shell shock, combat fatigue, flashback, combat psychosis, PTSD—
how do I bring the thousand-yard stare and scanning gaze
of trigger-edge alert back, back to focus on my face? On any face?

Naming the Monster

Young man, completely healthy until purple blotches
on his face doubled in a week, lungs whited out,
brain abscesses, oral fungus—on a vent on arrival,
dead the next day. He was the first we could not save

then a second, a third—
beautiful boys dead in days of exotic infections
sweating into skeletons, blind, confused, struggling
to breathe, kissed by purple sarcomas.

We wore masks and gloves, tried not to take fright
about what we did not know, stunned each morning
at the counts. San Francisco, 1980, no one knew
but suspicion fell on bathhouses, something

about being gay
although the soldiers insisted "not me"
preachers claimed divine retribution, Army regulations
demanded discharge to families that said "no,
we won't take him back"

antibiotics did not work and a blood splash, a needle stick
might be deadly, we added face shields, extra gloves
and a name—AIDS—which did not tame it, did not save one
gave no one comfort.

What To Say

I don't know what to say to the woman dying
in her eighty-ninth year—she tells me
to my making-conversation chatter
as I change the bandage—
"I told them I was homesick when I left
school, but there was a boy—
I let him kiss me once, but then he hit me
and held me down. . . he forced me. . .
I waited until the bruises
didn't show and went home,
but I kept thinking it showed somehow—
something in my face and I was scared.
When my period came, I thought, maybe
it was over, but it was never over.
When I lost all those babies I knew
it was me and when Joe cried,
I couldn't and the doctor said
I shouldn't try again and Joe
just stopped coming home."
I hold the roll of gauze above her leg
"You know, it's not your fault,
what that boy did." She shakes
her head and I unroll less briskly,
reach for what should come next.
"You never told?" She shakes
her head, I cup her heel
between both hands, think
of the moving seconds on the wall,
my waiting room outside.
"You should talk to someone," I say,
"it's not too late." Her eyes, pale blue, bright
with tears, meet mine.
She shakes her head and as she leaves,
redressed, she pats my hand.
"Thank you, Doctor" but now her guilt
is mine and when her niece says
at the funeral, "She was a difficult
person, hard to know, a little cold."
I don't know what to say.

Reconstruction

What do you say to the woman with the patchwork breast?
As you run fingers down fretwork ribs, along the bow of
 clavicle,
touch a purled knit of scar in her axilla, note tiny tattoos
 —blue,
unlike freckles, burns from the beams have faded into
 permanent tan.
Move aside the delicate gold chain with its single gray pearl
nestled in the throat hollow, her pulse a fast flutter.
Slip fingertips up anterior cervical paths to her jaw
then back down the knurled knobs of spine.
Bounce the stitched softball where her body layers
 firm denial
around the soft give of silicon and saline.
Sense your own breasts hanging heavy
in their sacks of lace and wire, armored, never safe
behind the white starch of coat, your embroidered name.
Remember gratitude for you both that this time,
no lumps, no need to add to the stitched puzzle
of chest and breast that isn't. What do you say
to the question in her eyes but "No lumps,
your breast is fine, nicely done reconstruction."

Swimming with Sharks

John says doctors have trouble
writing poems about *I don't know.*
Guilty culpability? Or maybe
the ingrained response to morning rounds
with its aggressive pimping for detail
and obscure diagnosis: *What! You can't tell me,*
from memory, the 27 causes of low sodium
and the last three days of this patient's hemoglobin?
We are taught that when you swim with sharks,
you must never bleed, that enticing sweat of fear
will bring an attack. Do not roll to show any soft
underbelly of uncertainty if you want
advancement in your field, stay silent and shift
to one side, if pinned give an unrelated fact.
It will take years to learn I don't know.
Decades for *I am sorry.*

She Says *Pneumonia, But Not Too Bad*

and even through the phone I hear tiny crackles in her breath.
She tells me *nine hours of tests and they sent me home, no fever today*
but it's hard to walk across the house, then spells azithromycin,

tells me she still plans to go to the party tomorrow night.
Doctor daughter collects more facts: blood tests, x-ray, O2 sat;
measuring concern against office schedules and ticket costs.

She has never liked to acknowledge "Mother," for years signs
letters *Jenny*. She says *I have a name. I'm more than meals,*
vacuuming, laundry and making beds.

But of six billion people in the world, she is the only one
I will ever call Mother. When I tell her this she begins to sign
her brief notes "Mom," sometimes adds a little arrowed heart.

I tell her that I love her, will keep my cell phone on. At my window
a hummingbird hovers, sips nectar from honeysuckle; the garden
is lush and weedy from recent rain. She says *I love you, too.*

We disconnect. For a long moment I listen to the hum of wings,
the harsh caw of crows overhead and from a neighbor's yard,
where the pine leans more each year, a chainsaw crackle starts.

Hunger

The window brightens from black to gray, no clear
transition of night to day as rain drizzles down still,
even the jays seem to know there will be no break
and crowd the feeder, hunger-pushed to shove in,
scattering seed to sparrows who wait below
or perch in draggled balls of wet fluff on the sill.

On this side of the window my cat crouches
twitches the tip of his tail, makes a soft chirrup.
I have heard the same sound more loudly and deep
from a tiger at the zoo when the keeper appears
with his tray of bloody meat. This cat
is too well-fed to need the tiny mouthfuls of flesh
twittering outside, but I thank the window for glass.

I could make the same sound as I think about my day,
hungry for my share: for a cup of hot tea and time to watch
rain and birds and cat. But the clock ticks on
and there are people drinking their own morning cups,
gathering their worries, little lists of need for me
to explain, reassure, write prescriptions for a pill
that will cure only the curable things.

Could I prescribe birds, seed and rain? Prescribe a cat
watching restrained by a window of fragile glass?
Instead, I fill the cat's bowl, measure out a cupful of seed,
gather white coat and keys, open my door and begin.

Hummingbird Feeder in October .

The nectar in my feeder may encourage
some to stay when they should fly
to southern climates where abundant

blooms will feed them and no freeze will stop
the rapid flutters of a tiny heart.
Put away the bottle or agree to vigilance:

keep the nectar filled and fresh no matter
darkness in the morning, fatigue when it's late,
rain and cold that keeps me near the fire

when I'm home after too many hours of clinic
caring for infinite needs: the woman alone
as cancer closes in, a mother locked in grief,

a man who struggles to keep sober, the suicidal girl –
no way to cut away pain, no cure in pills;
just nectar-drops of hope, a sweetness of belief,
as I make my hummingbird bargain.

Non Nocere

"Don't miss the important lesson," Daddy says,
as I pack the VW bug setting off for medical school.
"Which lesson?" I ask, counting boxes.
"The one that will kill someone if you miss it."
Fifty years later I still feel ice run
through me on that hot summer day—
the same fear as I stand beside a bed, hear alarms,
watch the green trace of heartbeat go flat.
The shiver as Mr. C. says, "Please, Doc, just kill me."
or when the daughter pleads, "Please,
you need to save her" and I say, "I can't,"
while I want to say "maybe…" "we could try…"
The old woman, tiny and curled, her mouth an O
of desert cave where dust puffs out with every breath
and the snap of her bone as I try, not gently enough,
to move her arm. So many ghosts
to be exorcised somehow.
So there are red zinnias for Harry
and foxgloves for Shirley, a persimmon tree
for Pam who would never save herself
and would not let anyone else try,
a hummingbird feeder for sweet Mrs. D,
a lemon tree for the horse that keeps Stephanie alive
years past what her oncologist predicts.
My garden of remembered faces —
Some days, enough.

The Sign Says

do not feed bread
to ducks   unnatural
nutrition for creatures meant
for weeds and small crustaceans
hidden in bottom muck

but the splendid mallards,
emerald gleams in early sun,
their frantic noisy joy
at my few crusts,
rescues me today.

For Want of a Gene

For Scarlet

For want of a gene a protein is lost
For want of a protein a neuron dissolves
For want of a neuron a muscle grows weak
For want of a muscle a baby can't walk

We cheer pink, cheetah-print leg braces
We wish for girlish happiness
And a killer fashion sense
We wish for sleekness and strength
We wish, like a cheetah, she could run
Faster than a missing gene

The Sound of Falling

Think of a sound: ripe pumpkin
dropped to concrete. Imagine
slick slippers, tile floor—

The ER intern grins *Squashed squash,*
a little blood clot—she'll be fine
and I remember a time I thought
sophisticated to say the same.

But you have lost marigolds,
Thailand and long division,
the last two weeks flattened
with a few ruffled folds of brain.

Now your rear flap untied,
you shuffle slow-mo to the john
rubber-soled slippers squeak
as they stick in the groove of last week,
and you ask for the tenth time today—

tell me again what went wrong

Falling

little difference between flying and falling
an instant untethered to earth, forward stumble
to flight and a second of suspension before gravity
reasserts and the earth reaches to smack you
back into dust. You will remember a vision of rock
trail, slick serpentine stones, a flash of your face
to that path and choice: dried rattlesnake grass
whispering to one side—*here, you can fall here,*
then whomp of a fist to your chest, mashed-out breath,
tumble and roll, roots to ribs, become a gasping fish
pain arrives as time stretches, elastic
sketched throb of blood as it spills into sealed spaces
wheeze of air trembling just out of reach, slow reach
and wiggle to find what moves and what won't
double vision of self-as-it-was and self-broken
as pieces scatter, reform.

Double Vision: Daughter/ Doctor

Daughter sits beside his bed remembering fever
when she was five and he sat her in a tub
to shiver down the thermometer,
reading *Horton Hears a Who*
until his hand on her brow said cool enough,
and wrapped her in a towel and carried her to bed.

Daughter wants the numbers down, wants
her father to wake up and talk about his golf game,
his plans for a new red car.
She tries to stay out of the way
when nurses come to turn and measure.

When he moans in pain she jumps, says *Dad*
do you need a shot for pain?
indecisive about calling a nurse.
Doctor sits beside his bed watching numbers
bounce and surge, knowing
too many permutations of disaster.

Doctor tries to hover visible, not intrusive,
wishing extra diligence into the nurses.
She is fluent in translation when doctors visit
saying *Fevers are not unexpected postop…*
meaning, *We don't know why…*
When he moans again, she jumps to find
the green button of the morphine pump
and since it is midnight and he should sleep, she pushes it.

Shoes

Sarge survived WWII, the South Pacific but 30 years
of cheap PX cigarettes brought cancer to his tongue.
He told me about snipers in palm trees while I drew blood
and fumbled two tries to start a line, I said the Army paid
for medical school and I would wear a uniform soon. He said,
"Godamn, I'll have to salute you." In 1976 his only chance
              —cut it out—
soon and radical. The senior surgeon described his plan—
remove half his tongue, jawbone and the muscles in his neck

Like a soldier, Sarge marched off to his battle,
but no one told him how weakened tissue can break loose—
turn him into a fountain, blood arching from his mouth
to the wall-clock across the room. Me, a bambi-student,
my short white coat clanking with penlights and hammers, ran.
In his room the resident grabbed my hand and jammed it
into his neck "Keep pressure there while I set the OR up"
then he ran as the intern sprinted to the blood bank
for everything they had. I said nonsense things: "Sarge,
you hang in there, you're doing great." He moved his lips
but whatever he needed to say was lost as his eyes roved,
then settled, pupils slowly dilating when I ran beside his bed
trying hard not to lose my grip. At the OR door, the resident,
scrubbed and sterile, reached in to take my place "Let go now.

Go home. Get some sleep, Come in after morning rounds."
then retreated with the gurney. A nurse was waiting:
wet towel, clean scrubs and two bottles of peroxide.
My once-white coat went into a bag, she said peroxide
was better than bleach but cold water first. I walked the
   November night
to my apartment and, two showers later, left my coat soaking
   in the tub.
The clothes and underwear went in the garbage with an apology
   to Sarge.
But the rules said leather shoes and skirts. Earth shoes releaved
my aching spine—light tan and expensive, no money in my budget
for another pair and peroxide did not work on leather.
An early morning trip to the 7-11 for a bottle of dark brown polish—
three coats covered the blotchy stains.

The intern said, "The Sergeant didn't make it," and we turned
to a lecture
on structures of the neck and the relative success of radical dissection.
Sometime after Christmas I found a sale and bought black leather
shoes.
It is odd how a memory hides for decades then jumps out, vivid,
impossible
when my ER nurses debate clogs or sneakers and Barbara
says she loves
her Crocs because they are so easy to hose off. And Sarge
was back again,
trying hard to send his final message as I walked for months
in his blood.

Expectant

We argued most over "expectant" – the soldiers so broken
that they would likely die but will tie up hours and personnel—
best left in a quiet corner, given morphine if they moaned.

Practice triage, our group of novice Army doctors
prepared for a future battlefield, hypothetical disasters.
The orthopedic resident was quiet, as we read each history
of injury, decided where each soldier went: minor patches—
like X-rays and a splint or a burn small enough to wrap
we took care of at the triage station.

Some we marked as "urgent", sent immediately
for surgery, to cut out bullets, pick shrapnel, sew
the punctures, amputate the mangled leg.

After we marked off the last imagined wounded,
the ortho resident said: "In Vietnam, I was shot
through the neck, assigned Expectant but stayed alive.
Fourteen hours later, a surgeon looked again and tried.
I don't remember air-evac, the early days state-side,
a blur of hospitals and surgeries, recovery very slow.
They said I was too old to be a doctor and maybe so,
but here I am."

II

Red Silk

Little in this world is pure pleasure. Maybe
the empty swing still dangling from the old oak.

Memory of a body pumping through space, stretching
to kick weightless blue, the joy of release, of flying through
breathless to thump on grass, a somersault into green.

Even as we die, life calls us to be a child again: bodies
becoming small and frail, minds simplified into delight
at the pattern of light reflected on the wall, the purr
of stroked cat, hummingbird hunger.

Hairless and soft, in cotton gowns washed to translucence,
we curl back into sleep in our cots protected
from falling by the raised steel rail.

We live in a culture where death is shunned. I think
we believe that ignoring them makes them go away,
but silence only makes them ugly. Matias Viegener

The gong, the ceremony of its ringing, the breaking
of silence creates silence.

Have you heard the old Irish tale that says that bards
are made by killing a red bull, taking its skin
and sewing a man inside? Left in darkness for three days
he emerges with the gift of poetry. Or he goes mad.

Death is not the worst thing that can happen to you.

Aspen trees and coral reefs are biologically immortal.
They are dying.

Three days in the hospital was $58,000.

In the Army, a silk camisole under
the camouflage fatigues saved my life.

Suppleness only exists if there is resistance. Suppleness
allows us to be intimate. Jane Hirshfield

Despair is a land-locked lake where no one lives,
the shore rimmed in salt. This image too pretty
for that place sealed against joy, where hope
is a sound pitched beyond hearing, where a day may
stretch for years, too painful to remain alive.

For years I lived in the last house before night.
I left the last month deposit behind.

Thirty years ago there was a woman who survived
the jump from the Bridge. She kept saying "no, don't, please"
as I punctured her veins. Later she thanked me. Later still
her car was found abandoned at Vista Point.

For years my drive across the Bridge was a coin toss.

In Florence, for one week I woke with each day unplanned.
Drinking wine at the Piazzale Michelangelo I watched
the city light itself at dusk. This was something like happiness.

Can I be homesick for a place I have never lived? Maybe
it was a place I saw once through a car window
as we drove the Texas panhandle in July in a car
without air or hope of rescue.

Did the old explorers feel exhilaration when they drew
upon the shores of home? Or just exhaustion?

Cadair Idris, a mountain in Wales; if you sleep there
for a night, you will awaken changed
into a poet. Or you will go mad.

So many poets are mad, or alcoholic or addicted
that it must be considered an occupational hazard.
Suicide may be seen as career progression for a poet.

*Persistent allodynia, which is pain resulting from a non-painful
stimulus such as a light touch, is a common characteristic
of neuropathic pain… persists long after the initiating event has resolved.*
Principles of Effective Pain Management at the End of Life

*Pain has an element of blank/ it cannot recollect/ when it began /
or if there were/ a day when it was not.* Emily Dickinson

Bodhisattva, do you regret your choice? said the voice in my head.
Can't you read the signs?

Miracle is the liquid in the cup lifting past the lip
in a quivering stasis. One more drop and all spills over.

A phenomenon of molecular attraction, surface tension
is often mistaken for miracle.

I have always been a rocket child on a trajectory of doubt.

I walked back to the fork where Mystic and Scientist parted,
where Good Girl screamed "Fuck it" and Poet sat down to wait.

The miracle was that years later Poet was still there
and no bull hides were required.

Sometimes too much of a good thing
is wonderful. Mae West

Sedona, with sandstone cliffs in more colors of red
than there are names, has a chapel carved into rock
high above the valley floor. It's a good place to light
candles. Something ought to be listening with all that red.

"Travel in expectation" is what the fortune cookie said.
I travelled with two GPS apps speaking different accents.
Sometimes the same directions, sometimes different
but somehow I got to where I needed to be.

Be complete in each thing. Put all you are
Into the least of your acts. Fernando Pessoa

An old man leans up the path with thin, deliberate legs.
Shorts bell out with each step. Curving forward to the hill
like a figure from a scroll drawn in ink and mist,
he rises higher and is gone.

Ilya carved his name into the varnished pine
of the bridge: a bear-boy with pocketknife claws.
When he is an old man will he remember the places
he's marked with his name? Will this feel like happiness?

The Coconino Forest is a forest without trees, a forest
of saguaro standing at gunpoint, a forest of creeks
and washes without water, a forest of sandstone
pillars the color of old blood.

I believe in winged-ness: in hummingbirds
and dragonflies, in the seeds of red maple twirling
like little hearts, in the miracle of lift coefficient.

The masseuse sweeps her hands down my neck to the tender
muscles of my scapula, says "You've been flying
hard, your wings are tired."

"In a quarter mile turn right to your destination" says
the cool female voice. The voice of the British butler
tells me "Continue straight ahead to Schnebly Road."

A roadrunner sprints along the middle.
I love Road Runner with his sassy "beep-beep" running
off cliffs, moving so fast and with conviction that he keeps going
through air. And Wile E., following just fine until he looks down
and believes in the fall so that he does.

The alchemy of sand and fire and breath is glass.
Gold added to the melt makes the purest red.

It is hard to be depressed when you wear
red silk against your skin.

III

Aubade

I remember Sunday mornings when hospital rounds
started late and I could awaken to the clock of sun
striped across the bedroom wall — early light of May
a rosy stain of color to your face, asleep,
worry lines unfurled into a younger you
for all the early silver to your hair, your lower lip
gentled, waiting for my wake-up kiss.
But I loved to watch you sleeping curled
against my hip, sleepy murmured protest,
blanket-burrowed resistance to the mirrored
dawn-light blinkered in your eyes, pulling you
from sleep to fractious day, I watched the return
of creased discontent as you tucked away
the boy so kissable and I took up my own armor for the day.

I Deliver Bad News

from the starch of my white armor
across a moat of polished oak.
You balance between an indrawn gasp
and grunt of pain. Myself, I'd as soon
not be here. I could drown
in the terror on your face as you look
into places I don't want to go.
I'd like to drop the news fast and cold,
close this play on opening night and run.
We might try this out as comedy—
The good news: you are going to die,
but neither of us could wear the baggy pants.
My nervous actor pleads *Come on, kids*
put on a show, things will work out swell.
Supporting hope against the odds is hard,
harder still to hold the silence,
the pleading of your need.

Fluent in Metaphor

You tell me about a pain and I wait.
Pain is an animal mostly, toothy,
sometimes slithery and scaled
as it slides through your gut.

Pain is never a rabbit, although
a heart may be a rabbit,
leaping startled from brush
across an open plain.

Your pain gnaws, wakes you
at 3 AM to pace. I wait
for you to name it in a story
about a brother with an ulcer
or a friend dead from pancreatic cancer.

If I translate incorrectly
you will remain un-healed
for all my pills to block acid,
despite pink pictures I show
of your colon, gleaming
un-polyped and un-cancered.

I would tell you that your body
is a swan, graceful and strong,
returning when it can to a place
of health and balance.

But, swans bring Ireland in
with starry night skys of Coole
or Zeus arrives in a clap of wings
and your 3AM pacing will resume
as you puzzle out my translation.

A storm is a bull, a boat is a wish
or maybe a bull is a storm
and a storm is a friend bringing word:
there is an end to drought.

Go To Where It Bleeds

When the cops arrived, the father met them
with butane and a knife while the ones he loved
flared incendiary, screaming *nononono*

into one long syllable of pain as the blue flames
flicked up bodies, burning skin, hair, muscle,
the boy's footed flannel pajamas

with bright dinosaurs melting
into flesh. Almost still a baby and never
going to be a child. He whimpered

when the morphine lightened as we scrubbed
and picked the bits of char. The nurse crooning *baby,*
you're gonna be OK, you're doing fine — for the boy,

for me, the shiny intern with my new blue scrubs,
my shaking hands holding a scalpel to scrape free
the sticking bits. My resident trying for coolness

says *you got to get to where it bleeds*,
offers me a swipe of VapoRub to block the smell
of a charred body. His mother in the burn unit

downtown, no news on Dad, no explanation.
Baby moans and the nurse edges up
the morphine as his hair pulls off in melted mats,

ear curled and blanched. *Probably going to lose the ear*
the attending surgeon says as he begins to plan his grafts.
He says *Poor kid it will to be bad* but I never know

as I go to lectures on grading burns, calculate
body surface area and percentage of survival
and the problem of scars: how they harden,

contract into a rigid shell. No one mentions
years of pain or a life lived with a terrible truth
that love is a porous shield, impossible for some.

Baby Boy, can you twist a life around this night,
twist it hard into a scar, leave it to mark the lintel
of your years ahead? Can you see the sinuous
scarred beauty of your precious life?

Words Beyond Words

Words beyond words: your sudden wince of pain,
your indrawn breath, the tightening of your throat,
the way your shoulders rise, defensive with some strain.
You sit with tiny rockings of your body like a boat.

If you were I lion I would check your paw for a thorn.
If you were a horse I'd check your saddle for a burr.
You say nothing's wrong, you are just a little worn
from not sleeping lately and isn't there a pill to blur

the edges just a bit, some advertisement on TV?
A jotted scrip would be a quick fix; to sound how deep
the unspoken river of your troubles might be—
a slower passage as the minute hand creeps.

True healing comes from stories: the telling, the listen.
"Tell me," I say and see your tears begin to glisten.

Night Call

If you are in need and it is midnight,
if I leave my bed for the cold darkness,
if I stumble on the step, drive yawning to the ER,
if the light is fluorescent and numbing
and there are cries of despair from the next bed,
I will not resent more than a little
my dream forever gone, not curse you
for the warmth cooling beneath my quilt.
I will not hold you accountable
for the missing hour of sleep.
I will love the crescent moon, the sudden deer
and hustling skunk on my street as I return.
I will love this midnight world.
I will love my calling.
I will love your need.

Remission

The calla lilies have gone
from tapered candles of prayer
to gratitude. Their ivory cups spill

the light of slanted sun.
In a pool of warmth, the cat sleeps,
his fur is haloed gold. The vet says,

"In remission, maybe another year."
What needs doing now
can wait as I pluck a tangerine,

peel the fragrant rind,
scattered in scraps of orange
around my feet, pull apart

the sections, eat
tart and sweet in equal parts.
I watch the sun slide down the sky

as the cat moves to my lap.
Over my shoulder the pale disc
of moon rises toward the night

Tell the Bees

For Paula

We must tell the bees that she is gone.
She kept no skeps to drape in black
but her gardens covered the town—
bloom-spilling baskets from lamp poles,
green paths up summer-straw hills,
her house with flowery skirts for all seasons:
azaleas, roses, sweet-smelling stock,
peonies, asters and mums, quiet
cool corners of pine, trickled water
for music, wind through the boughs.
She loved abundance, needed
to give laughter and love, scattered
her friendships like seed.
She kept no hive in her garden,
but the bees know a queen.
We must tell them so they can grieve.

What We Don't Know

A handful of treasures: unexpected healings,
sudden certainties like when I hold sobbing Marcy,
know she will be the statistic who lives, give
a sybil-like promise for a year of suffering, and a long life.
Decades later she sends Christmas pictures
of the newest great-grand-baby.

Franny whose rage screams through years of grief
as I sit beside her on the crinkled exam-table paper,
my nurse runs in, terrified at the sound. Her husband
was so sure he had cancer no one could find,
but he found the hidden gun and she takes so long
to live again while I learn the dance progresses
as it will and comfort only takes where allowed.

Lisa, single mom, lung cancer spread, says *I died before*
when my heart stopped, a good place, but my daughter
was too young and I had a choice, came back
but she's grown now, so don't do that again.
The chill on my neck rises hair. She dies at home,
her daughter cries, then lives, fully loved.

Barbara, cancer spread, stays alive on belief
in water blessed by the Virgin at Knock. She asks me
how to live ready to die, *What's my purpose?*
My answer, without thought: *Maybe you teach doctors*
what we don't know, remind us of things beyond numbers.
Seven years later, at her death, she leaves me bottles of water
for someone who might ask. Most I give away, one I keep.

Of Love and Electronic Health Records

Once, and sometimes still, I love the space
of my exam room with its ritual of question
and listen, the whiff of ancient fires and drums,
where love is necessary to the cure.
Now Dr. J tells me to cultivate a love of algorithms,
the cunning codes for human condition:
compression of the brain (G93.5),
injury caused by falling (W19). Could anyone
love an EHR? Its freezes and myriad clicks?

Mine causes a love for sleep, upright
in my roller chair, drool on my chin, hand to mouse
and nnnnnnnnnnnnnnnnnnnnnnnnnnnnnnnnnnnn—
nnnnnnnnnnnnnnnnnnnnnnnnnnnnnnnnnnnnnnn—
nnnnnnnnnnnn scrolling a pixillated screen.

My day: Barry, the nerdy boy with his sketchbook
full of heroes, Betty who talks to her plants,
Sharon who lives in her car because a shelter
will not let her keep her dog, the unknown
woman with her sign I saw slink
through rain at the freeway verge—
stakes are high and the fall is long.

How does love reach across a digital divide
to fill cracks, the fine craquelure of grief,
porcelain mended with threads of gold
more beautiful and fine, if more fragile,
in a world that forgets we need to give love,
how unspent it will choke our melancholy song?

The ICU Nurse Sang

The ICU nurse sang and held one hand of the nameless man—
told me to hold the other, reminded me to breathe when he did not,
and tears, she said, were fine— contrary to the professor who sneered
at mine, at my first death, told me to hide moist eyes in paperwork.
But with this man, found dying and alone, we stood on either side,
him between, silenced alarms, screens left dark, while her soft lullaby
filled the hollow places and the man lay quiet until he died.

The Drug Salesman Leaves a Bag of Fortune Cookies in the Break Room

You are the controller of your destiny
Cellophane envoi, 3 dozen fortunes
brought to you by Paxil. Drug-rep bribery,
cookie back-scratch, *prescriptions,*
please, in return. Newly approved
for depression with generalized anxiety disorder.
Call it GAD, *please sign for samples.*

You will soon be crossing the great waters
David says it's the plastic, all the healthy bottled
water leaching cancer-causing molecules
with tiny, feral grins bringing on the plague:
Marian and Doris and Sally and Marie,
more than two a month: a lump, a breast,
chemo takes their hair. I'm back to drinking Bon Tempe.

Your pursuit of happiness is an endless trail of good humor and pleasure
Choleric, melancholic, phlegmatic, sanguine.
Bile brings stones and leeches are back in style.
Lizard spit keeps me uncurdled, less sweet.
I should have bought stock in your drug.
If I start to flick my tongue, throw nets.

You will have good luck in your personal affair
News clippings from the ex: in Japan
the oldest recorded woman can't be found,
her family promises to return seven years of
pension checks. His hand-written note—
3 lines: "The company renewed my contract.
I guess I'm staying here. Did the cat die yet?"

You will be unusually successful in business
One day's office mail: 5 insurance forms, 2 disability claims,
1 school sports exam, 30 prescription refills, 4 pounds of trash,
1 journal gets read first, cover by Degas—*his first*
ballerina explains M. Therese Southgate, MD
who out of love presents each week art and erudition;
fortified bread around the filling of avian flu, the latest drug,
and proof: fish won't hold off age, and wrinkles can kill
(some) insistent on their removal.

You are gifted in many ways
San Francisco Fortune Cookie Company
3 dozen pieces, approximate count.
Flour, sugar, salt, partially hydrogenated vegetable oil
Natural flavorings, serving size: one cookie.
No calories in luck.

Pray for what you want, but work for the things you need
I am not good at flocks and sheep
get shorn or eaten. Father Tom says
I think too much but, still, a crucifix
is an instrument of torture,
and, even smiling, Mary is looking sad.
Are you happy, Father Tom?

There is no substitute for hard work
More bars and a little shit-kicking music
in my twenties might have helped.
Attitude! Black leather, maybe, or a jacket
of purple silk. My libretto says *"The Blues"*
and I still don't know the tune.

A faithful friend is a strong defense
My body is the lady in the lamplight
humming "*Carmen*." She will drop me
to my knees if I am rude,
but, kindly; she will smile as she flamencos
small fiery steps along my spine.

Now is the time to resolve all unfinished business
the man in 3406 is waxy with death but it won't be real
until I listen, slow count, stare into his starless night,
pupils wide and unflinching at the mylar fish swimming
the ceiling above his head, announce aloud the time
"one thirty-seven." I always pick odd numbers,
write in careful black

Very soon, and in pleasant company

Red Hill Dissolving

The community passes petitions
to "Save Red Hill", collects change
in jars by the registers at Andronico's
and the Union 76, but with each rain

the cracks widen and the streets
run with clay. In the ICU machines
push air in and out for another week,
colored liquids drip into your body

and then flow away. Through the window
I watch the creek redden and rise
with January rain and one great white heron
stalks the bank trailing feathers stained

with mud. We have forgotten: not everything
wants to be saved. There is a weird beauty
in the twirl of white oleander
blossoms floating down the red flood.

The Body Keeps Its Own Refrains

Lessons repeated   then again
to be helpless   to wait
a body battles to die   or tries to live
rhythms of   breathe and gasp
slick of skin sweated   with fever or pain
how eyes can roam   unseeing
pass sightless   over the best beloved
Or fix for hours   on a ceiling crack
as if some answer   was there
entire   formed   dimensional clay
molecules of breath   passed through a lung
crackling with humors   always mysterious
for all the microscope slides   memorized
landmarks   of flesh   paths of drugs
mystery of bloodflow   turns of DNA
the body keeps its own refrains

Madonna of Tomato Soup

Renaissance Madonna, her face floats
in candlelight—luminous porcelain of calcined
bone and palest clay. Her collar bones

mark a ridge beneath her knitted shirt.
She spoons small sips of thick soup—
tomato and cream, says *Delicious,* and

I'm glad to be out of the hospital.
A neighbor, I've met her here before
and Mirabelle, her fat beagle

slowly creeps to my lap.
She tells me *I'm lucky, I have a twin,*
a donor match for marrow.

I want to believe her languid motion,
her erect spine are grace, not the rampage
of wild cells softening bones to pain.

I admire her bravura—aubergine scarf
pulled close to her sculptured skull, a twist
of gold and green silk at the rim

tied into a flower over one ear.
She lifts a bite of birthday cake
and I see she has no eyebrows.

I've heard prayers help, a friend
has a friend—Diné, he has prayed
with sage smoke and eagle feathers.

After dinner, we walk the dark street,
Mirabelle keeping steady pace. I offer
a ride, but she says *I like to walk when I can.*

All week I am haunted by her face—at the beach,
a wave-peeled stick, bleached ivory on dark sand,
looks like a clavicle, the green silk at my neck,

a beagle passes by on a leash,
and I need to pray but for her or for me?

Song of Dark and Windy Nights

The Golden Gate has learned to sing in hums and moans—
a siren song from Baker Beach to Conzelman Road.
The new lightweight walk thrums in wind and
after 75 years, 2000 jumps recorded, they are adding nets
in hope of saving some, but this year a record has been set.
The bridge with its fogs and sparkling views—a magnet
for those lost in darkness and in despair.
1980: a girl pulled from the water beneath the bridge
brought to my ER to our tsunami of saviors,
we cut away her clothes, wrapped her in hot air,
punctured her with tubes while she murmured.
"No. Don't. Please just let me go." Surgeons took her,
took her torn spleen and kidney, pinned steel in broken bones
then sent her to a hospital downtown.
Regular reports said she was talking to psychiatrists,
taking pills for depression, physical therapy had her walking
with a cane, eventually discharged her home.
They found her car abandoned at Vista Point.
And now they've taught the Bridge to sing.

Why I Seldom Sing

My voice, lost to laryngitis, needs rest
for weeks, shifts into whisper, rasps
and squeaks into sudden fits.
Unconscious in the years of medicine,
I find a lower tone, assure my colleagues
and my patients I am not a frivolous girl,
can be trusted with a life, my orders
followed without question and now
a speech therapist holds my throat
through prolonged *eeeee* until my breath
gives out— she says my voice is lost
to too much talk, lost to camouflage—
though a deeper pitch gives gravitas
it scars the cords into silence.
I've broken through walls to gain my calling
and the breaking took my voice.

My Mother's Hands

small and soft, knobby fingers
brown-spotted from the sun she loves
fine veins thread beneath thin skin
bruised from the search for blood
gold and sparkle from many rings
I ask her if she is in pain, she squeezes
my hand once, says "No, I'm fine,"
coughs and rolls to her side still holding on
until the nurse comes to check.

Mercy

For Camille

The nurse insisted I must come,
must "address a feeding tube"
And I thought of a conversation
with a rubber hose, "Monsieur,
let me introduce you to Mrs. C,
she is one hundred and nine
and does not eat
in clear violation of Title 22."

To lose weight is a fineable offense,
easily prevented by a tube in the nose.
She did nicely on brie
and baguettes — nourishment
for any Gaelic soul until one too many falls
brought her from her home
to the mercy of a proper dietician
and a healthy diet of blandly, low-fat food.
Mrs. C ate little, then less. "So,"

I said, "we're worried." And she began:
The quality of mercy is not strain'd
it droppeth as the gentle rain from heaven
upon the place beneath, it is twice blest…
quoting each line to the end …*to mitigate*
the justice of your plea. She breathed.
The world needs more Portias,
are you a going to be a Portia?

She got no tube.
She did not eat.
She died in a week:
her death, a gentle rain.

Contrails

A line of vapor along the western sky—straight with drips
like a gooey sweet, marshmallow frosting slipping down,
or an edge of roof with icicles; angled up across the blue.
a plume of white dropped by an ostrich of enormous size.
I am a contrail connoisseur like when I was eight; the Colorado
sky was high and nearly enameled blue, trails of passing planes
rare and lost in piles of cumulus. On a summer afternoon
sometimes Daddy for a treat would join an hour of finding shapes:
elephant, clown, crocodile-becoming-horses or spouting whales.
Now Daddy sits to watch the evening sky as clouds boil up
above Pikes Peak. He drinks a glass of wine, talks to Mom,
looks for signs in the shapes he sees: a heart, an aspen leaf,
maybe a little dog. I ask him how he knows
which ones are her. He says, "I know."

It Has Been a Year

For my mother

Eastern clouds brighten
into gray haze,
Mt Tam a suggestion
sketched in ink and fog.
My phone rattles a question
from a friend, I reply
a single word – *fine.*
Extra blanket, a cup of Earl Grey
I cannot warm. It has been a year
and, still, you are dead.

Yahrzeit Moon

Full moon at 3 AM, bright and round,
ducking through fast-moving cloud,
wind wuthers through the chimney,
moans across the downspouts, rattles trees,

the house a creaky ship
in storm-frothed seas, across the valley –
scattered lights: porch lamps, streetlights,
windows, a car turns up a twisted drive.

Neil posts it is his mother's yahrzeit.
He asks for prayers. Minyans are uncertain
in a time of viral plague, as we huddle away
from smiles and touch, the comforts ritual brings.

My mother died three years ago,
I add a prayer for her, I can't manage Hebrew —
but read aloud the English words:
May there be abundant peace from heaven …

Are the ones on the far hillside awake
to listen to the wind? Are they well?
Are they afraid? And who listens to us all?

I Want To Hold You In My Arms

…in thanks, in gratitude, in comfort,
for friendship, for the trust you have given,
for the freedom to make mistakes.
But your children gather around your bed—
your daughter holds one hand and your husband
holds the other and I must be something firm
and upright for them to lean on.
So I turn off the monitor where light traces
the stutters of your heart, stop the beeps
of alarm coming from the vent and settle
for holding one toe.

ACKNOWLEDGMENTS

The following poems were originally published:
Brats (Finishing Line Press) "Night Call"
Marin Poetry Center Anthology, "Red Hill Dissolving"
Mom Egg Review, "Yahrzeit Moon"
Naugatuck River Review, "Reconstruction," "Song for Dark and Windy Nights"
Purrfect Poems: Poems In Support of Stafford Cat Rescue, "Remission"
Tell Me Again: Poems and Prose from The Healing Art of Writing 2012, "Mercy" "Words Without Words"
The Western Journal of Medicine, "I Deliver Bad News"
Tiny Tim Review: "For Want of a Gene"
Touch: Journal of Healing, "Hunger"

A special thank you to Octavio Quintanilla, whose artwork appears on the front cover.

Short Title: "Cats sleeping on the rooftops."

Full Title:
"I can still see the cats sleeping on the rooftops / and see the moon's snout touch you / through the windowpane / of that old building / where we learned that love was older / than all / of our darkness."

Octavio Quintanilla's work on Instagram.
Instagram: @writeroctavioquintanilla
https://www.instagram.com/writeroctavioquintanilla/

NOTES

Page 2: Triage – a system of rapidly assessing an illness or injury and assigning urgency. In a situation of many patients and limited resources, it includes deciding how to allocate care to the most people.

Page 4: PTSD – Post Traumatic Stress Disorder. Baghdad by the Bay is a nickname for San Francisco, where Letterman Army Hospital was located. Fleet Week is the yearly Navy turnover in San Francisco Bay. The Blue Angels are the Navy precision flying team.

Page 5: Vent is an abbreviation for a ventilator. Sarcoma is cancer that shows as purple splotches on the skin, often seen in people with AIDS.

Page 8: Surgeons are often called sharks by other specialties in the hospital. Pimping is aggressive questioning from a senior doctor to a trainee doctor meant to test knowledge and also humiliate the student.

Page 9: Azithromycin is an antibiotic. O2 sat is a measure of the oxygen level in the blood.

Page 12: Non nocere—do no harm, from the Hippocratic Oath.

Pages 18-19: PX is the Post Exchange—a military department store. OR is the operating room.

Page 20: Orthopedic residents are doctors in their second through fourth year of training after medical school. Air-evac means evacuating or removing an injured soldier from the battlefield by air to a hospital in an area not involved in combat. State-side is the United States.

Page 22-25: Camouflage fatigues are Army uniforms marked with an irregular pattern of green and brown.

Page 31-32: Grafts are skin grafts: skin taken from an unburned area placed over the burn to cover it and help it heal.

Page 33: Scrip is a written prescription.

Page 35: Remission is the apparent absence of cancer after treatment. Cats get cancers too.

Page 36: There is an old superstition that when there is a death in the home, the beehives should be draped in black cloth. And the bees told gently of the death, or the bees will leave in grief.

Page 38: EHR is an Electronic Health Record.

Page 39: ICU is an Intensive Care Unit.

Page 45: Baker Beach is just south of the Golden Gate Bridge. The Bridge has a steady number of people who jump to their death and a few who survive. In the last few years, nets along the walkways were added, and the Bridge has picked up a humming vibration in strong wind.

Page 48: Title 22 is California law governing nursing homes. The quality of mercy… is from Portia's speech in *The Merchant of Venice* by Mr. William Shakespeare.

Page 51: Yahrzeit (anniversary in Yiddish). On the anniversary of a loved one's death, Jews burn a candle and say prayers for them.

ABOUT THE AUTHOR

Catharine Clark-Sayles grew up in a military family, went to medical school, and became an Army doctor, followed by a private internal medicine and geriatrics practice. In 2019 she completed an MFA in poetry and narrative medicine at the Dominican University of California. Tebot Bach Press published previous collections, *One Breath* and *Lifeboat,* and a chapbook, *Brats*, published by Finishing Line Press. *The Telling, The Listening* is her fourth book drawn from forty-five years of medical practice.

Typefaces Used

GARAMOND - Garamond
PERPETUA TILTING MT

www.ingramcontent.com/pod-product-compliance
Lightning Source LLC
LaVergne TN
LVHW051018080826
845145LV00009B/2682
9781955194181